Jamaican Herbal Remedies

A Beginner's Guide with a 7-Step Action Plan and Sample Recipes

mf

copyright © 2025 Isadora Kwon

All rights reserved No part of this book may be reproduced, or stored in a retrieval system, or transmitted in any form or by any means, electronic, mechanical, photocopying, recording, or otherwise, without express written permission of the publisher.

Disclaimer

By reading this disclaimer, you are accepting the terms of the disclaimer in full. If you disagree with this disclaimer, please do not read the guide.

All of the content within this guide is provided for informational and educational purposes only, and should not be accepted as independent medical or other professional advice. The author is not a doctor, physician, nurse, mental health provider, or registered nutritionist/dietician. Therefore, using and reading this guide does not establish any form of a physician-patient relationship.

Always consult with a physician or another qualified health provider with any issues or questions you might have regarding any sort of medical condition. Do not ever disregard any qualified professional medical advice or delay seeking that advice because of anything you have read in this guide. The information in this guide is not intended to be any sort of medical advice and should not be used in lieu of any medical advice by a licensed and qualified medical professional.

The information in this guide has been compiled from a variety of known sources. However, the author cannot attest to or guarantee the accuracy of each source and thus should not be held liable for any errors or omissions.

You acknowledge that the publisher of this guide will not be held liable for any loss or damage of any kind incurred as a result of this guide or the reliance on any information provided within this guide. You acknowledge and agree that you assume all risk and responsibility for any action you undertake in response to the information in this guide.

Using this guide does not guarantee any particular result (e.g., weight loss or a cure). By reading this guide, you acknowledge that there are no guarantees to any specific outcome or results you can expect.

All product names, diet plans, or names used in this guide are for identification purposes only and are the property of their respective owners. The use of these names does not imply endorsement. All other trademarks cited herein are the property of their respective owners.

Where applicable, this guide is not intended to be a substitute for the original work of this diet plan and is, at most, a supplement to the original work for this diet plan and never a direct substitute. This guide is a personal expression of the facts of that diet plan.

Where applicable, persons shown in the cover images are stock photography models and the publisher has obtained the rights to use the images through license agreements with third-party stock image companies.

Table of Contents

Introduction   7
All About Jamaican Herbal Medicine   9
    Overview of Jamaican Herbal Traditions   9
    Importance and Benefits of Herbal Remedies   10
    Safety Considerations and Guidelines   11
Essential Jamaican Herbs and Their Uses   13
    Detailed Profiles of Key Herbs   13
Preparing Herbal Remedies at Home   21
    Methods for Creating Teas, Tinctures, and Poultices   21
    Dosage Guidelines and Storage Practices   26
    Tools and Equipment Needed   27
7-Step Action Plan to Incorporate Herbal Remedies   30
    Step 1: Identifying Personal Health Goals   30
    Step 2: Selecting Appropriate Herbs   34
    Step 3: Sourcing Quality Ingredients   37
    Step 4: Preparing Remedies   42
    Step 5: Integrating Remedies into Daily Routine   47
    Step 6: Monitoring Progress and Adjusting   52
    Step 7: Adjusting and Customizing the Approach   57
Sample Recipes for Common Ailments   62
    Herbal Tea Blends for Digestion and Relaxation   63
    Topical Applications for Skin Health   68
    Remedies for Respiratory Support   73
Integrating Herbal Remedies with Modern Medicine   78
    Understanding Interactions and Contraindications   78
    Communicating with Healthcare Providers   80
    Combining Traditional and Contemporary Approaches   82
Growing Your Own Medicinal Herbs   84
    Tips for Starting a Home Herb Garden   84

Soil, Climate, and Care Requirements	86
Harvesting and Preserving Techniques	88
Resources and Further Reading	**91**
Recommended Books	91
Trusted Websites	93
Local and Online Suppliers	94
Workshops and Courses on Herbal Medicine	95
Conclusion	**97**
FAQs	**100**
References and Helpful Links	**103**

Introduction

Jamaican herbal medicine is a vibrant tapestry of culture, history, and nature woven together over generations. This traditional practice draws from the island's abundant biodiversity and the combined knowledge of African, European, and indigenous roots.

With its unique approach to natural healing, Jamaican herbal medicine has become an invaluable resource for addressing common ailments, promoting well-being, and maintaining connection to ancestral traditions.

The richness of this tradition lies in its focus on using readily available herbs to create remedies that are effective, accessible, and deeply respectful of nature. From the calming properties of soursop leaves to the immune-boosting power of turmeric, these remedies go beyond symptomatic relief to nurture the body, mind, and spirit. They offer a holistic approach to health, often emphasizing prevention through regular use of herbal tonics, teas, and poultices.

In this guide, we will talk about the following:

- All About Jamaican Herbal Medicine
- Essential Jamaican Herbs and Their Uses
- Preparing Herbal Remedies at Home
- 7-Step Action Plan to Incorporate Herbal Remedies
- Sample Recipes for Common Ailments
- Integrating Herbal Remedies with Modern Medicine

Keep reading to learn more about the fascinating world of Jamaican herbal medicine and how you can incorporate it into your life for optimal health and well-being. With a deeper understanding of this ancient practice, you will not only gain valuable knowledge but also gain a greater appreciation for the natural wonders that surround us.

All About Jamaican Herbal Medicine

Jamaican herbal medicine has a rich history deeply rooted in the island's culture and natural resources. This traditional practice is a blend of African, European, and indigenous knowledge, reflecting the diverse heritage of the Jamaican people. Known for its reliance on locally available plants, Jamaican herbal medicine continues to play an essential role in natural health and wellness, offering alternative paths to healing and prevention.

Overview of Jamaican Herbal Traditions

The foundation of Jamaican herbal medicine lies in the relationship between the people and their environment. With Jamaica's abundant biodiversity, over 50% of the plants found on the island are believed to have medicinal properties. Traditionally, herbalists, known as "bush doctors," have served as key figures in the community, using extensive knowledge of plants to create remedies for various health conditions.

Many of these practices were passed down orally from generation to generation, ensuring the survival of valuable knowledge. Remedies often include teas, poultices, tinctures, and baths derived from plants such as soursop, cerasee, guinea hen weed, and turmeric. Each of these herbs carries unique benefits and forms part of the holistic approach Jamaican herbal medicine offers, treating not just symptoms but aiming to restore balance to the entire body.

Importance and Benefits of Herbal Remedies

Herbal remedies are significant in Jamaican culture for their accessibility, affordability, and effectiveness. For many, they represent a sustainable approach to health care, relying on all-natural ingredients from the surrounding environment. They also bridge generational and cultural gaps, offering a sense of continuity and connection to ancestral traditions.

The benefits of herbal remedies are wide-ranging. Soursop leaves, for example, are commonly used to ease anxiety and promote sleep, while cerasee tea is praised for its detoxifying and blood-purifying qualities. Ginger, another staple, is well-known for soothing nausea and aiding digestion. Jamaican herbal medicine's focus on using whole, natural ingredients also means remedies often come with fewer side effects compared to synthetic drugs.

Additionally, herbal traditions emphasize prevention just as much as treatment. Regular consumption of herbal teas or tonics can boost immunity, enhance energy levels, and promote overall well-being. This preventive approach aligns with a broader trend toward holistic health, making Jamaican herbal medicine appealing to those seeking natural alternatives in today's wellness landscape.

Safety Considerations and Guidelines

While Jamaican herbal remedies offer numerous benefits, it is important to approach them with care and consideration. Not all herbs are suitable for every individual, and incorrect preparation or dosage can pose health risks. Traditional herbalists highly value the importance of proper identification and treatment expertise, which underscores the need for informed use.

It is advisable for individuals to consult qualified herbal practitioners before using unfamiliar plants, particularly if they have pre-existing medical conditions or take prescription medications. Pregnant and breastfeeding individuals should also exercise caution, as certain herbs may not be safe in these situations.

Additionally, sourcing high-quality herbs is crucial. Using organic and ethically harvested herbs ensures greater potency and minimizes exposure to harmful substances like pesticides. Following recommended preparations, such as proper boiling times and correct concentrations for teas, can further enhance safety and effectiveness.

Jamaican herbal medicine showcases the strong connection between culture, history, and nature. Its traditions, health benefits, and holistic approach make it valuable for modern wellness practices. By respecting these remedies, individuals can benefit from Jamaica's diverse plant life while prioritizing safety and balance in their health journey.

Essential Jamaican Herbs and Their Uses

Jamaica's lush, tropical terrain is home to a diverse range of herbs with powerful medicinal properties. These plants have earned a central place in traditional Jamaican healing practices, often used to address common ailments and promote overall wellness. Below, we'll explore five key herbs, detailing their profiles, health benefits, applications, and practical guidance for cultivation or sourcing.

Detailed Profiles of Key Herbs

1. **Moringa (Moringa oleifera)**

   Moringa, known as the "Miracle Tree," is one of the most nutrient-dense plants on the planet. With its ability to thrive in warm climates, it grows abundantly across Jamaica and is used frequently in teas, powders, tinctures, and food recipes. All parts of the tree – leaves, seeds, pods, and roots – are valued for their health benefits.

Medicinal Properties

- Packed with vitamins (A, C, E) and essential minerals like calcium and potassium.
- Contains amino acids that support muscle and tissue repair.
- High levels of antioxidants help combat oxidative stress, supporting cellular health.

Common Applications

- *Teas*: Dried moringa leaves are steeped to create a tea that supports immune function and energy levels.
- *Capsules or Powders*: Moringa powder is consumed as a supplement to boost nutrition.
- *Skin Care*: The oil extracted from moringa seeds is commonly used in skincare to reduce inflammation and keep the skin hydrated.

Cultivation and Sourcing Tips

Moringa thrives in sunny, warm climates and tolerates drought, making it ideal for Jamaica's weather. Grow it from seeds or cuttings in loose, well-draining soil. It's a fast-growing plant and can be harvested within months of planting. If sourcing, look for organic or ethically grown moringa products to ensure optimal quality.

2. Turmeric (Curcuma longa)

Famous for its vibrant orange-yellow color, turmeric has long been celebrated for its culinary and medicinal uses. Known in Jamaica as a "root of life," it is frequently included in teas, tonics, and topical remedies.

Medicinal Properties

- Rich in curcumin, a compound with potent anti-inflammatory and antioxidant properties.
- Aids in reducing joint pain and stiffness.
- Acts as a natural antibacterial and supports a healthy liver.

Common Applications

- *Turmeric Tea*: Fresh or dried turmeric, boiled with ginger and honey, is a popular remedy for colds and digestive troubles.
- *Golden Milk*: Turmeric is mixed with milk (or plant-based alternatives), cinnamon, and black pepper to create a soothing nighttime drink.
- *Topical Pastes*: Turmeric mixed with water or aloe vera is applied to wounds or inflamed skin areas to speed up healing.

Cultivation and Sourcing Tips

Turmeric grows best in warm, humid environments. Plant rhizomes (root pieces) in moist, well-drained soil and partial shade. It requires consistent watering but should not be waterlogged. Harvest the rhizomes after 8–10 months of growth when they're vibrant and aromatic. When sourcing turmeric, prioritize fresh roots or organic ground turmeric.

3. Cerasee (Momordica charantia)

Cerasee, also known as bitter melon vine, is a staple in Jamaican households. Despite its characteristic bitterness, it is one of the most trusted herbs for detoxification and rejuvenation.

Medicinal Properties

- A natural blood cleanser that supports detoxification.
- Helps regulate blood sugar levels, making it beneficial for diabetic patients.
- Contains anti-inflammatory and antimicrobial compounds that support immune health.

Common Applications

- **Detoxification Tea**: Cerasee leaves and vines are boiled to create a tea that cleanses the blood and supports digestive health.

- **Baths**: The boiled leaves are often added to baths to soothe skin irritations.
- **Topical Washes**: The extract can be applied to cuts, insect bites, or rashes for its antibacterial benefits.

Cultivation and Sourcing Tips

Cerasee is a hardy, fast-growing vine that thrives in sunny environments with freely draining soil. It can easily climb fences or trellises. If wild-sourcing, be mindful of sustainability; ensure that the plant population is being preserved. For dried herbs, choose a reputable supplier who avoids the use of unnatural chemicals.

4. **Ginger (Zingiber officinale)**

Ginger is indispensable in Jamaican homes, not only for its culinary uses but also as a go-to remedy for a variety of conditions. Known for its warming and invigorating properties, it is often paired with other herbs to enhance their effects.

Medicinal Properties

- Stimulates digestion and alleviates nausea.
- Contains gingerol, a compound with anti-inflammatory and antioxidant effects.

- Supports respiratory health by reducing congestion and soothing sore throats.

Common Applications

- *Ginger Tea*: Boiled slices of fresh ginger root, often sweetened with honey, is the most common preparation for colds and nausea.
- *Compresses*: Warm ginger paste is applied to relieve joint pain or muscle stiffness.
- *Culinary Use*: Fresh grated ginger is widely used in Caribbean cooking to flavor dishes while boosting their health benefits.

Cultivation and Sourcing Tips

Ginger grows best in warm climates with filtered sunlight. Plant rhizomes in nutrient-rich, well-draining soil. Keep the soil moist but avoid waterlogging. Ginger can be harvested after about 8–10 months or when the leaves begin to yellow. For freshness, purchase whole ginger roots and store them in a cool, dry place.

5. **Soursop (Annona muricata)**

Soursop leaves, fruit, and seeds are widely used in Jamaican herbal medicine. This tropical plant has gained international attention for its potential health benefits.

Medicinal Properties

- Contains acetogenins, which may contribute to its potential anti-cancer properties (though more human studies are needed).
- Promotes relaxation and sleep due to its natural sedative effects.
- Supports immune system health with its high vitamin C content.

Common Applications

- *Soursop Tea*: Leaves are steeped in hot water to create a calming tea that supports healthy sleep patterns.
- *Juice*: The fruit's pulp is blended to make a refreshing juice rich in antioxidants and energy-boosting nutrients.
- *Topical Poultices*: Crushed soursop leaves are applied to alleviate skin issues or inflammation.

Cultivation and Sourcing Tips

Soursop trees grow well in tropical climates with fertile, well-draining soil. They require full sunlight and regular watering but are relatively low-maintenance once established. Leaves should be harvested directly from healthy trees and used fresh or dried for preservation. If sourcing the dried leaves, ensure they are from reputable growers to confirm their authenticity.

Cultivating your own herbs is an excellent way to ensure a fresh, high-quality supply while reducing reliance on commercial sources. However, not everyone has the space or time to grow their own. For purchases, always purchase from reliable vendors who prioritize ethical and organic practices. Look for herbs that are non-GMO and free from artificial additives.

Learning about these key Jamaican herbs brings you closer to using traditional herbal medicine in daily life. Each plant offers unique benefits, whether you're brewing teas, making pastes, or adding them to your diet for preventative care.

Preparing Herbal Remedies at Home

Jamaican herbal medicine isn't just about the plants themselves; it's also about how they're used. By preparing your own remedies at home, you can ensure the quality and freshness of the herbs while crafting solutions tailored to your needs.

This chapter offers practical guidance to help you get started, whether you're steeping a soothing tea, crafting a restorative salve, or preserving herbs for long-term use.

Methods for Creating Teas, Tinctures, and Poultices

Mastering these three traditional preparation methods is a great starting point for anyone exploring herbal remedies. Each method serves a different purpose, ranging from internal healing to external applications.

1. **Herbal Teas (Infusions and Decoctions)**

   Herbal teas are one of the simplest and most common ways to consume medicinal plants. Depending on the herb, teas can serve as an immune booster, digestive aid, or even a sleep remedy.

   Infusions are used for delicate plant parts like leaves or flowers, while ***decoctions*** are better suited for tougher materials such as roots, barks, or stems.

   Steps to Make an Infusion:

   - *Prepare the Ingredients*: Use 1–2 teaspoons of dried herbs or 2–3 teaspoons of fresh herbs per cup of water.
   - *Boil the Water*: Bring water to a rolling boil, then pour it over the herbs in a heat-resistant container.
   - *Steep*: Cover the container to trap the essential oils and steep the mixture for 10–15 minutes for dried herbs, or 5–10 minutes for fresh herbs.
   - *Strain and Serve*: Use a fine strainer or a cheesecloth to separate the liquid from the herbs. Sweeten with honey or add a slice of lemon if desired.

   Steps to Make a Decoction:

- ***Prepare the Herbs***: Measure about 1 tablespoon of dried herb or root per cup of water.
- ***Simmer***: Combine the herbs and water in a pot and bring to a gentle boil. Reduce heat and simmer uncovered for 20–30 minutes, depending on the hardness of the plant material.
- ***Strain***: Remove from heat and strain the liquid. This method is ideal for herbs like ginger or turmeric root.

Additional Tips:

- Always use non-reactive cookware like stainless steel or glass when preparing remedies.
- To preserve the medicinal qualities, avoid over-boiling herbs.

2. **Tinctures**

Tinctures are potent herbal extracts preserved in alcohol or glycerin, which make them easy to store and use long-term. They're particularly useful for herbs that lose potency quickly when dried.

Steps to Make a Tincture:

Choose Your Herb: Use high-quality dried or fresh herbs, chopped to increase surface area.

Combine Ingredients: Place the herbs in a glass jar, filling it about halfway. Pour a high-proof alcohol like vodka (or non-alcohol alternatives like vegetable glycerin for alcohol-free tinctures) over the herbs until the jar is full.

Seal and Store: Seal the jar tightly and store it in a cool, dark place for 4–6 weeks. Shake the jar daily to ensure even extraction.

Strain and Bottle: After the steeping period, strain the mixture through a cheesecloth or fine mesh strainer. Transfer the liquid into dark glass dropper bottles for storage.

Dosage and Usage:

Tinctures are concentrated, so use them sparingly. A typical dosage is 1–2 ml (20–40 drops) diluted in water or tea, taken 1–3 times daily depending on the herb and desired effect.

3. **Poultices**

Poultices are external applications made by mashing herbs into a paste and applying them to the skin to treat inflammation, wounds, or pain.

Steps to Make a Poultice:

- **_Prepare the Herbs_**: Crush fresh herbs using a mortar and pestle or rehydrate dried herbs with warm water.
- **_Form a Paste_**: Mix the herbs with water, honey, or a natural oil (like coconut oil) until it forms a thick paste.
- **_Apply_**: Spread the paste evenly over a clean piece of cloth or gauze. Place the cloth over the affected area, ensuring the paste is in direct contact with the skin.
- **_Secure_**: Use a bandage or wrap to hold the cloth in place. Leave the poultice on for 20–30 minutes, or up to an hour for deeper relief.
- **_Cleanse_**: Remove the poultice and rinse the area with lukewarm water.

Common Herbs for Poultices:

- **Turmeric** for inflammation
- **Aloe Vera** for burns and cuts
- **Peppermint** for muscle aches

Tips for Success:

- Test a small area first to check for allergic reactions.
- Poultices should be freshly made for every use.

Dosage Guidelines and Storage Practices

Proper dosing is essential to ensure the remedies are both safe and effective. Storage practices also play a crucial role in maintaining the potency of your preparations.

Dosage Guidelines

1. ***Start Small***: Beginners should always start with the smallest recommended dosage and gradually increase only if the body responds well.
2. ***Herb-Specific Recommendations***: Each herb has its own safe dosage range; consult resources or professionals for guidance. For example, cerasee tea should not be consumed daily for extended periods due to its detoxifying intensity.
3. ***Listen to Your Body***: If you experience unusual side effects, discontinue use and consult a healthcare provider.
4. ***General Measures***:
   - Teas: 1–3 cups per day depending on the herb.
   - Tinctures: 1–2 ml diluted in water, up to 3 times daily.
   - Poultices: Apply for short durations (max 1 hour) to avoid skin irritation.

Storage Practices

1. ***Teas***: Consume freshly made. Store unused tea in the refrigerator and consume within 24 hours.

2. ***Tinctures***: Store in dark glass bottles away from heat or light; these can last up to two years.
3. ***Dried Herbs***: Keep them in airtight containers in a cool, dark place. Properly stored, dried herbs retain potency for 12–18 months.
4. ***Fresh Herbs***: Wrap loosely in a damp cloth and refrigerate. Use within a week for maximum potency.

Tools and Equipment Needed

Having the right tools ensures that your herbal preparations are effective and easy to make. Here's a list of essential items for your herbal toolkit:

1. ***Mason Jars***: Essential for creating infusions, decoctions, and tinctures. Their airtight seal keeps your preparations fresh, and their transparency allows you to monitor the process easily.
2. ***Fine Mesh Strainer or Cheesecloth***: Perfect for separating plant material from liquids, ensuring smooth, debris-free infusions and tinctures. Cheesecloth is ideal for finer straining, while a mesh strainer works well for coarser materials.
3. ***Mortar and Pestle***: A traditional tool for crushing fresh herbs into pastes or powders, releasing their natural oils and maximizing their potency. It's a must-have for anyone working with raw plant materials.

4. ***Saucepan or Teapot***: Use these for brewing herbal teas or decoctions. A sturdy saucepan allows slow simmering, while a teapot is perfect for steeping delicate herbal blends.
5. ***Glass Dropper Bottles***: Ideal for storing tinctures or potent extracts. The dropper allows precise dosing, making them great for herbal remedies or essential oils.
6. ***Kitchen Scale***: A tool for accurately measuring herbs by weight. Precision is key in herbal preparations, and a digital scale ensures consistency across your recipes.
7. ***Dark Storage Containers***: Essential for preserving dried herbs and protecting them from light exposure, which can degrade potency over time. Amber or cobalt-colored glass jars are great options for long-term storage.

Additional Nice-to-Have Tools:

- Herb scissors for cutting fresh herbs.
- Thermometer to monitor water temperature for delicate herbs.
- Labels and markers to document preparation dates and contents.

By mastering these preparation methods and following the dosage and storage guidelines, you'll have everything you need to create safe, effective herbal remedies at home. With the right tools and a little practice, you can confidently tailor your remedies to suit your unique health needs while maintaining the rich traditions of Jamaican herbal medicine.

7-Step Action Plan to Incorporate Herbal Remedies

Herbal remedies can be a valuable addition to achieving a healthier lifestyle, but using them effectively requires a thoughtful and informed approach. This chapter will walk you through a 7-step action plan to seamlessly incorporate herbal remedies into your daily routine.

Step 1: Identifying Personal Health Goals

Your journey with herbal remedies starts with understanding what you truly want to achieve. When you can clearly define your health goals, you're setting yourself up for success right from the beginning. This isn't just about identifying problems you want to fix, but also about optimizing your overall well-being. Here's how you can dig deeper to find out what matters most to you:

Reflect on How You Feel Right Now

Take a moment to reflect on your overall health. Are there aspects of your life that feel unbalanced? Perhaps you've been experiencing frequent headaches, fatigue, or difficulty sleeping. Or maybe you feel generally healthy but want to boost your immunity or better manage stress. Consider both your physical and emotional well-being as you assess where improvements might be needed.

Ask yourself:

- Do I feel energized throughout the day, or am I often fatigued?
- Are there minor issues, like bloating or frequent colds, that I've been ignoring?
- Am I managing stress effectively, or do I feel overwhelmed?
- Is my overall mood where I want it to be?

Writing your answers down can help you organize your thoughts and pinpoint your focus areas.

Prioritize What Matters Most

Once you have a list of health concerns or areas for improvement, prioritize them. After all, it's easier to tackle one or two issues at a time. For instance, if you've been dealing with regular digestive discomfort, that might be your top priority. If stress has been taking a toll on your mental health, it could be your starting point. Establishing a clear order of priorities keeps you focused and avoids spreading your efforts too thin.

Visualize Your Ideal Outcome

Think about what success looks like for you. If your goal is reducing stress, imagine feeling calm and in control no matter the situation. If you want to support your immunity, envision staying healthy through flu season without interruptions. Having a mental picture of your desired results can keep you motivated as you begin incorporating herbal remedies.

Break Your Goals into Smaller Focus Areas

Big goals can often feel overwhelming, but breaking them into smaller, specific objectives can make them more manageable. For instance:

- If your overarching goal is "better digestion," smaller objectives might include reducing bloating, preventing heartburn, or encouraging regular bowel movements.
- If you aim to improve sleep, you might break it down into falling asleep quicker, staying asleep through the night, and waking up refreshed.

Small, actionable goals allow you to track progress more easily and build confidence along the way.

Ask for Feedback from Your Body and Mind

Pay close attention to how your body and mind respond throughout the day. Keeping a simple health journal for a week or two can offer valuable insights into your well-being. Record details like energy levels, mood changes, sleep quality, and recurring symptoms. Identifying patterns can uncover hidden issues you might not have linked to your health goals.

For example:

- Do your energy levels dip after lunch? This could signal a dietary change rather than just a need for more sleep.
- Are tension headaches popping up after stressful meetings? Stress relief herbs like passionflower or valerian could be on your radar.

Set Clear and Achievable Goals

Now that you've explored your health in detail, phrase each goal in a way that is clear and actionable. Instead of saying, "I want to feel better," try something like:

- "I want to calm my nerves without relying on sugary snacks or caffeine."
- "I want to breathe easier and reduce my allergy symptoms."
- "I want to improve my slow digestion through natural support."

These well-defined goals act like a roadmap as you move to the next steps of this herbal remedy plan.

Health is dynamic and evolves with age, environment, and lifestyle. Setting clear goals is important, but staying flexible ensures they align with your changing needs. Reflecting and prioritizing thoughtfully helps create a personalized approach, especially when exploring herbal remedies. Listen to yourself to move forward confidently.

Step 2: Selecting Appropriate Herbs

Now that you've identified your health goals, it's time to choose the right herbs to support them. Picking the right herbs takes research, personal insight, and sometimes professional advice. By making thoughtful choices, you can ensure your remedies are safe, effective, and meet your needs. Follow these steps to decide with confidence.

1. **Match Herbs to Your Health Goals**

    Start by looking for herbs that are known to support the specific goals you've outlined. For example:

    - If you want to improve digestion, herbs like ginger, fennel, or peppermint may address issues like bloating, nausea, or sluggish digestion.
    - If stress or anxiety is your focus, calming herbs like chamomile, passionflower, or ashwagandha are worth exploring.
    - For immunity, you might consider elderberry, echinacea, or garlic due to their immune-boosting and antiviral properties.

Using reliable herb guides, wellness books, or trusted online resources can give you valuable insights into how each plant works. Keep a notebook where you can jot down potential options and their benefits.

2. **Understand Herb Properties and Uses**

Go beyond the surface understanding of an herb. For each one you're considering, learn about its specific properties and how it addresses your particular concerns. Some herbs are known for their calming effects, while others are energizing, detoxifying, or nourishing. It's also worth understanding:

- *The part of the plant used* (e.g., roots, flowers, leaves, or seeds) since this influences how it's prepared and what benefits it provides.
- *Common preparations* (e.g., teas, tinctures, powders, or capsules) and which form might work best for your lifestyle.
- *Duration of use* (short-term versus long-term) to avoid any potential side effects from overuse.

3. **Consider Safety and Side Effects**

Not all herbs are for everyone, so it's crucial to think about your unique body and health situation. When evaluating herbs, consider:

- *Allergies or sensitivities*: Does the herb come from a plant family that you might react to? For

example, people allergic to ragweed might also react to chamomile.
- *Medications you are taking*: Herbs like St. John's Wort can interact with prescription drugs, including birth control and antidepressants.
- *Existing health conditions*: Certain herbs may amplify conditions. For instance, licorice root should be used cautiously by those with high blood pressure.
- *Life stage*: If you're pregnant, breastfeeding, or providing for a child, research which herbs are safe for these stages.
- Research any potential contraindications carefully, and when in doubt, seek professional guidance.

4. **Start Small and Simple**

When beginning with herbs, avoid overwhelming yourself by selecting too many all at once. Choose one or two primary herbs to focus on while you're still learning. This way, it's easier to track how your body responds without confusing variables. For example:

- If your goal is better sleep, start with one calming herb like valerian root or chamomile before trying complex blends.

- If digestion is your focus, choose either ginger or fennel rather than mixing several herbs immediately.

Starting small allows you to fine-tune your herbal practice while building confidence and knowledge.

5. **Opt for High-Quality Information**

    Be selective about where you get your advice. Authentic herbal traditions, qualified herbalists, naturopaths, or well-reviewed herbal guides are excellent sources. Avoid falling for exaggerated claims or relying on unverified online forums. Focus on credible, evidence-based resources that back up their information with traditional wisdom or scientific research.

6. **Consult an Expert**

    Consulting a certified herbalist or integrative healthcare provider can help you choose safe, effective herbs tailored to your needs. With patience and curiosity, explore alternatives if one doesn't work, and thoughtfully incorporate herbal remedies for better health and well-being.

Step 3: Sourcing Quality Ingredients

Finding high-quality herbs is one of the most important steps in ensuring the effectiveness and safety of your herbal remedies. Not all herbs are created equal, and taking the time to source premium, uncontaminated ingredients will give you the best chance of achieving your health goals. Here's how you can confidently choose herbs that are potent and trustworthy.

1. Choose Reputable Suppliers

Start by identifying suppliers that have a strong reputation for providing quality products. Whether you're purchasing online, at a local health store, or from a farmers' market, do your homework. Look for sellers who prioritize transparency about their sourcing practices. Here are some things to consider:

- Does the supplier provide information about where their herbs are grown?
- Do they share details about how the herbs are harvested, dried, and packaged?
- Are they willing to answer your questions about their products?

Trustworthy suppliers often have reviews or testimonials from satisfied customers. Take a moment to read them to spot any red flags or consistent praise.

2. Look for Organic Certifications

Certified organic herbs are grown without synthetic pesticides, herbicides, or fertilizers, which might linger as harmful residues on the plants. When possible, choose organic ingredients to reduce your exposure to these chemicals and support more sustainable agricultural practices. Look for certifications such as:

- USDA Organic
- EU Organic
- Organic by other trusted national agencies

Keep in mind that some smaller producers may not have official certifications but still follow organic growing practices. If this is the case, don't hesitate to ask questions about their farming methods.

3. Check for Quality Indicators

When purchasing dried herbs, there are a few physical characteristics that can help you assess their quality:

- *Color*: High-quality dried herbs typically maintain some of their natural color. For example, peppermint leaves should appear green rather than brown or dull, and turmeric root should have a vibrant orange hue.
- *Aroma*: Freshly dried herbs should have a strong, identifiable aroma. If the smell is faint or non-existent, the herb may have lost its potency.
- *Texture*: Crumbly or overly dry herbs may be too old. Look for pliability in dried leaves,

flowers, or roots, which indicates proper processing and storage.

This is particularly important if you're purchasing in bulk or from self-serve bins in health food stores.

4. Avoid Additives and Fillers

Some commercially available herbal products may contain additives, fillers, or artificial preservatives. Always read the ingredient label carefully. Pure herbal products should list only the herb and perhaps a natural preservation method (like alcohol in tinctures). Products with long ingredient lists or unfamiliar names may be less effective or even harmful.

5. Support Sustainable and Ethical Practices

When sourcing herbs, think about sustainability. Overharvesting of wild plants can lead to environmental degradation and endanger native species. Here's how you can choose herbs responsibly:

- Opt for herbs that are cultivated rather than wild-harvested unless sustainably sourced.
- Look for suppliers that prioritize eco-friendly farming practices.
- Consider using herbs that are native to your region, as they tend to be more sustainable and can support local ecosystems.

Additionally, research whether the suppliers treat their farmers fairly, especially for herbs sourced internationally. Ethical sourcing ensures that workers and communities involved in cultivation are treated with respect and compensated properly.

6. Grow Your Own Herbs

If you have the space and interest, growing your own herbs can be an excellent way to guarantee quality and freshness. Start with beginner-friendly herbs like basil, mint, or thyme, which grow well in pots or small garden spaces. By cultivating your own ingredients, you'll know exactly where they come from and how they've been handled. Plus, it's an opportunity to connect more deeply with your remedies.

7. Inspect Packaging and Storage Conditions

Proper storage is key to preserving potency. When buying pre-packaged herbs, avoid products stored in clear plastic or exposed to direct sunlight, as these factors degrade essential oils and active compounds. Instead, look for herbs packaged in airtight, opaque containers or resealable bags. If you're buying loose herbs in person, check that the storage bins are clean and the herbs are rotated regularly.

At home, store your herbs in a cool, dark, and dry location, in airtight containers, to retain their freshness.

8. **Test a Small Batch First**

    If you're trying a new supplier, start by ordering a small amount to assess quality. This allows you to test the aroma, color, and effectiveness of the herbs before committing to a larger purchase. Some reputable suppliers even offer sample-sized quantities so you can ensure they meet your standards.

9. **Build Relationships with Local Herbalists**

    Support local herbalists and small-scale growers for high-quality, sustainably sourced herbs while preserving herbal traditions. Prioritizing quality ensures safe, effective remedies that honor nature's healing properties and set the stage for confident preparation.

Step 4: Preparing Remedies

Preparation is a crucial step in the use of herbal remedies. It ensures that the healing properties of the herbs are extracted effectively and used in a way that aligns with your health goals. While the methods for creating teas, tinctures, and poultices have been covered previously, this step focuses on the importance of preparation, how to choose the right method, and tips for avoiding common mistakes.

The Importance of Preparation in Maximizing Effectiveness

Proper preparation of herbs is what transforms raw plants into powerful remedies. Without careful preparation, the potency and benefits of the herbs can be diminished. For instance:

- Boiling or steeping some herbs for the wrong amount of time can reduce their medicinal compounds or, in some cases, create unpleasant flavors that discourage use.
- Incorrect storage or handling during preparation can cause herbs to lose their freshness, rendering remedies less effective over time.

By dedicating attention to the preparation process, you can ensure that your remedies deliver the intended healing benefits. Proper preparation also allows you to adapt the strength, formulation, or quantity of herbs based on your personal needs.

Choosing the Right Preparation Method

Each preparation method serves a unique purpose depending on how the remedy will be used and what you want to achieve. Here's a breakdown to help you choose the most suitable method:

- *Teas and Infusions*: Ideal for addressing internal health concerns like digestion, stress relief, or hydration. Teas are gentle and often used for regular, sustained use.

- ***Tinctures***: Perfect when you need a more potent, concentrated remedy in smaller doses. They are great for chronic conditions or when portability and long shelf life are important.
- ***Poultices***: Used for external applications, particularly for skin issues, inflammation, or injuries. These remedies are targeted and fast-acting for localized relief.
- ***Infused Oils and Salves***: Recommended for skincare, muscle tension, or wounds. These are rich in soothing compounds and create a barrier that supports healing.
- ***Decoctions (boiled remedies)***: Suitable for dense or hard herbs like roots and bark, which require longer, stronger extractions to release active compounds.

Selecting the right method often depends on whether the remedy is meant for:

1. ***Internal Healing*** (soothing, nourishing, or detoxifying the body).
2. ***External Relief*** (addressing visible or topical concerns like rashes or bruises).

Tips for Ensuring Potency and Effectiveness

The way you handle and prepare your herbs greatly affects the potency of your remedies. Keep these tips in mind to create high-quality preparations:

1. *Use Fresh, Quality Herbs:*
   - Whenever possible, opt for fresh, organically grown herbs. If fresh herbs are unavailable, turn to high-quality dried herbs that retain their aroma and color.
   - Ensure herbs are stored in airtight containers away from heat and light.
2. *Follow Preparation Guidelines:* Each herb is unique and requires specific preparation techniques. For example:
   - Delicate flowers like chamomile need minimal heat or steeping time to avoid losing their active properties.
   - Hardy roots like ginger or turmeric benefit from longer or hotter preparation.
3. *Pay Attention to Ratios*: Using the right proportion of herb to liquid (or other extraction medium) is key. Overloading herbs may result in overly strong remedies, while using too little may dilute their effects.
4. *Handle with Care*:
   - Wash and dry herbs carefully to remove dirt without bruising delicate plants.

- Use non-reactive tools like glass or ceramic rather than metal, which can alter the flavor or composition of remedies.

5. ***Store Properly:***
    - Keep your prepared remedies in dark, airtight bottles to prevent exposure to light and air that can degrade their strength.
    - Label your containers clearly with the preparation date and any specific details about the remedy.

Common Mistakes to Avoid

Even with the best intentions, errors during preparation can reduce the quality or safety of herbal remedies. Be mindful of these common mistakes:

1. ***Using Herbs Without Research***: Not all herbs are safe for everyone. Some may interact with medications, while others may not be suitable for long-term use. Always research or consult a trusted source before working with unfamiliar herbs.
2. ***Incorrect Dosages***: Using too much or too little of an herb can either cause unwanted side effects or limit its effectiveness. Start with moderate amounts and adjust as needed while observing any changes in your body.
3. ***Contamination Risks***: Failing to clean tools, jars, or herb materials properly can introduce bacteria. Ensure

that all equipment is sterilized, especially for remedies like tinctures that are stored for long periods.
4. **Rushing the Process**: Many remedies, like tinctures or infused oils, take time to prepare. Trying to speed up the process may result in reduced potency. Patience is essential to extract the full healing properties of herbs.
5. ***Overlooking Quality Standards***: Old, faded, or poor-quality herbs won't yield good results. Be selective about your sources and avoid low-cost options that compromise freshness or quality.

Preparing herbal remedies requires intention and respect for the process. By carefully selecting methods and avoiding common mistakes, you can create effective remedies tailored to your needs. Combining traditional wisdom with attention to detail ensures confidence and care in your creations.

Step 5: Integrating Remedies into Daily Routine

The real magic of herbal remedies happens when they become part of your everyday life. A remedy isn't much help if it sits untouched in your cabinet, so the key is finding ways to seamlessly weave it into your routine. By making small adjustments and staying consistent, you can ensure you're taking full advantage of your herbs' benefits without feeling overwhelmed. Here's how to do it.

1. **Pair Remedies with Existing Habits**

   One of the easiest ways to integrate a new habit is to pair it with something you already do. For example:

   - Add your herbal tea to your morning ritual by sipping it alongside your breakfast or as you start your workday.
   - Take tinctures or capsules before brushing your teeth or preparing dinner, so it becomes second nature.
   - Apply herbal salves after your shower when moisturizing your skin is already part of your routine.

   By attaching herbal remedies to activities that are already familiar, you'll be less likely to forget them.

2. **Create Visual Reminders**

   Sometimes all you need is a little nudge to stay consistent. Keep your remedies visible and easily accessible:

   - Place your tinctures or capsules on the countertop or near your coffee maker.
   - Keep herbal teas where you usually store your mugs or favorite snacks.
   - Store salves and oils in your bathroom, where you can grab them as part of your skincare routine.

Strategic placement means your remedies are out of sight only when they don't need to be.

3. **Set a Schedule that Works for You**

Choose times of day that align with the purpose of each remedy. For example:

- Sleep aids like chamomile tea or valerian root are best taken in the evening to help you wind down.
- Energy-boosting herbs such as ginseng or ashwagandha might work better in the morning or around midday.
- Digestive support herbs like ginger or peppermint could be taken before meals to promote healthy digestion.

Stick to a consistent schedule so your body can get used to the benefits over time. You can even set alarms or reminders on your phone to help you stay on track during the first few weeks.

4. **Start Small and Build Gradually**

If you're new to herbal remedies, start with one or two remedies rather than trying to incorporate everything at once. For example, you might begin with an herbal tea each evening or a tincture twice a day. Once you've established these habits, you can gradually add more remedies as needed. This approach will prevent overwhelm and help you identify which remedies are working best for you.

5. **Make It Enjoyable**

Integrating herbal remedies shouldn't feel like a chore. Find ways to make the experience enjoyable:

- Add a slice of lemon or a drizzle of honey to your herbal tea for extra flavor.
- Use your remedies as an opportunity to pause and practice mindfulness. Savor the taste of your tea or the sensation of applying a calming salve.
- Create a cozy ritual around taking your remedies, like wrapping yourself in a blanket with your tea in hand or listening to relaxing music as you take your tincture.

When you look forward to the process, you're more likely to stick with it.

6. **Track Your Consistency**

Use a journal, habit tracker, or even a simple checklist to document your herbal remedy routine. Note the remedies you take, the time of day, and how you feel afterward. This doesn't just help you stay consistent; it also gives you valuable insight into what's working and what might need adjusting.

7. **Stay Flexible**

   Life happens, and some days may not go as planned. If you miss a dose or skip a remedy on busier days, don't stress. Herbal remedies are most effective when used consistently over time, but occasional lapses won't undo your progress. Focus on getting back into the groove when you can.

Example Routine Integration

To illustrate how remedies can fit into a typical day, here's an example schedule:

- *Morning*: Start the day with a cup of green tea infused with ashwagandha for energy and focus. Take your immune-boosting tincture after breakfast.
- *Afternoon*: Drink a digestive tea, like peppermint or fennel, after lunch to alleviate any bloating or discomfort.
- *Evening*: Use a lavender-infused oil to massage your temples, incorporating relaxation and aroma therapy into your wind-down time. Sip on chamomile tea about 30 minutes before bed.

Make your herbal remedy routine fit your lifestyle by staying flexible and listening to your body. Adjust formats or timing as needed to create a sustainable habit that supports your health goals. Once it feels natural, focus on tracking results and refining your approach.

Step 6: Monitoring Progress and Adjusting

Using herbal remedies takes time, and it's important to track how well they work for you. Monitoring progress helps you see what's improving, what needs adjusting, and how your body responds. The key is to stay consistent, observant, and open to changes. This ensures you're moving forward with purpose. Here's how to refine your herbal remedy routine.

1. **Keep a Detailed Journal**

    Tracking how you feel each day will give you valuable insights into how the remedies are impacting your health. Dedicate a notebook or digital app for journaling, and create a consistent routine for recording your progress.

    Include these details:

    - *What remedy you took*: List the herb, dose, and preparation method (tea, tincture, salve, etc.).
    - *When you took it*: Time of day can influence how remedies work, so record this too.
    - *How you felt before and after*: Note any physical, mental, or emotional changes you experience. For example, did chamomile tea

help you relax before bed? Did ginger relieve your stomach discomfort after lunch?

Additionally, track any reactions or side effects, like allergic responses or sensitivity. These notes will build a clear picture of what works best for you.

2. **Be Patient with Results**

Herbal remedies often work gradually, so give your body time to adjust. Some results, like lavender's calming effects, may appear quickly, while others, like improved digestion or immunity, can take weeks. Stay consistent and use them regularly for 4–6 weeks before evaluating. Herbal remedies focus on long-term balance, not quick fixes.

3. **Watch for Specific Changes**

Pay attention to how your symptoms change over time. Ask yourself:

- Is your energy level more stable throughout the day?
- Are you sleeping better after incorporating a bedtime remedy?
- Have you noticed improved digestion or reduced discomfort?
- Are your stress levels or mood changes less pronounced?

Tracking specific improvements builds motivation and helps identify the remedies contributing to these positive changes.

4. Adapt to Your Body's Signals

Each person responds differently to herbs, so it's critical to listen to your body's unique signals. If something doesn't feel right, don't hesitate to make adjustments. Here's how:

- *Tweak the Dosage*: Adjust the dose slightly up or down (within safe limits) and monitor the effects for better results.
- *Change the Preparation Method*: Tea might not provide the same results as a tincture or capsule. If one form doesn't seem effective, try another.
- *Adjust the Timing*: Some remedies work better when taken at certain times (e.g., energy-boosting herbs in the morning vs. calming teas in the evening).

Adaptability is key. Small changes can make a big difference in how remedies work for you.

5. Set Goals and Milestones

Having concrete goals will help you evaluate your progress. For example, if you're using herbs to improve digestion, your milestone might be less bloating or heartburn over a two-week span. Celebrate small wins, like fewer restless nights after using a calming remedy. These checkpoints will keep you motivated and give you a clear sense of direction.

6. Seek Input When Needed

You don't have to do this alone. If you're unsure about your progress or not seeing results, reach out for professional guidance. A certified herbalist, naturopath, or healthcare provider can:

- Offer personalized recommendations based on your symptoms and history.
- Suggest complementary remedies or adjustments.
- Help you identify potential interactions with medications or other supplements.

Sometimes expert advice can provide the clarity you need to fine-tune your routine.

7. Reevaluate Periodically

Herbal remedies should evolve with your changing needs. Every month or so, take time to reflect on your progress:

- Are your original health goals still relevant, or have they shifted?

- Have you resolved certain issues, but new ones emerged?
- Do you still enjoy using the remedies, or do they feel like a burden?

This evaluation process allows you to adjust your approach. For example, if your stress has improved but sleep remains an issue, you could reduce stress-focused remedies and explore new ones for sleep support.

8. Don't Overlook Setbacks

If you don't see the results you were expecting, don't view it as a failure. Instead, use it as an opportunity to learn. Common reasons for setbacks include:

- *Incorrect dosage or form*: Try adjusting how you're taking the remedy.
- *Timing issues*: Some herbs are more effective when used at certain times.
- *Underlying factors*: Sometimes, the issue you're addressing is just a symptom of a deeper condition that may require medical attention.

Make adjustments as needed and remind yourself that healing is a process.

Step 7: Adjusting and Customizing the Approach

Adjusting your herbal remedy routine is essential for achieving long-term wellness. Over time, your body's needs may change, and fine-tuning your approach ensures your remedies remain effective, safe, and aligned with your health goals. This step is all about flexibility and personalization.

Why Adjustments Are Necessary

Every individual responds uniquely to herbs. Factors like stress levels, seasonal changes, diet, or even life events can shift your body's requirements. What worked perfectly for you a few months ago might need adjusting to better fit your current condition. By observing your body's signals and being open to change, you can maximize the benefits of herbal remedies without wasting time or resources.

How to Make Adjustments:

1. *Change the Dose*

   Start small when trying a new herb and increase the amount gradually if needed. If you don't notice any improvement, slowly bump up the dose until it feels right for you (but stay within safe limits). On the other hand, if you feel uncomfortable or notice side effects like mild stomach troubles or drowsiness, scale the dose back.

Example: If your valerian tea isn't helping you sleep, try drinking a stronger brew or adding a second cup to your routine until you see results.

2. *Adjust the Timing*

When you take your remedies matters! Some herbs work better at specific times of the day:

- Take **energizing herbs** (like ginseng) in the morning to boost your energy for the day.
- Use **calming herbs** (like lavender or chamomile) in the evening to help you relax or sleep better.

Example: A cup of chamomile tea an hour before bed can help you unwind, while a ginseng tincture in the morning can kick-start your energy levels.

3. *Try a New Approach*

If you're not seeing results, it might be worth changing how you use a remedy. For example, if teas aren't working well for you, try a tincture or capsule instead. You can also experiment with new herb combinations to address multiple needs at once.

Example: If peppermint tea isn't easing digestion as much as you'd hoped, peppermint capsules might work better for you.

Reevaluate and Reflect Regularly

Reevaluation is a vital part of keeping your wellness plan in sync with your evolving needs. Set aside time every few weeks or months to check in with yourself and your progress.

Ask Yourself:

- *How Do I Feel Overall?:* Have your symptoms improved? Are you meeting your original health goals? For example, is your digestion better, or are you sleeping more soundly?
- *What's Working Well?:* Identify the remedies that are making a positive difference. Keep these as part of your routine and consider exploring similar herbs to build on the success.
- *What's Not Working?:* If certain remedies don't feel effective or enjoyable to use, adjust or replace them. No remedy works universally, and part of the process is finding what truly resonates with you.
- *Are There New Health Concerns?:* Life changes, stress, or aging can bring new challenges. Check if your health goals have shifted and explore remedies targeted to those new priorities.

Examples of Reevaluation in Practice:

- If stress-focused herbs like ashwagandha have helped you feel calmer, but you're still struggling with

fatigue, you might add energizing herbs like rhodiola or adaptogens for stamina.
- If a remedy is no longer helping as expected, consider pausing its use for a while. Your body can sometimes build tolerance to herbs, and taking breaks can make them effective again.

The Importance of Flexibility and Adaptability

Herbal remedies aren't one-size-fits-all, and what works today might need a different approach in the future. Flexibility allows you to personalize your wellness plan over time, ensuring it serves your unique goals and lifestyle.

- View Setbacks as Learning Opportunities: If a remedy doesn't work as intended, it's not a failure. Use it as a chance to understand your body better and adjust accordingly.
- Stay Patient: Herbal remedies often work gradually, so give them time before deciding to change course. Allow at least 4–6 weeks of regular use before drawing conclusions.
- Seek Guidance When Needed: If you're unsure about adjustments or aren't seeing the results you expect, consult an herbalist, naturopath, or healthcare professional. They can help pinpoint what's missing or offer alternative suggestions.

By fine-tuning dosages, altering timing, exploring new methods, and reflecting on your progress regularly, you'll create a flexible and sustainable approach to health. Adjusting your herbal routine ensures it grows with you, supporting your wellness in a way that feels personal, effective, and empowering.

Sample Recipes for Common Ailments

Jamaican herbs provide a treasure trove of natural remedies to tackle everyday health concerns. With five recipes across each category, you now have even more options to address digestive issues, promote relaxation, support skin health, and bolster respiratory well-being. Here are the detailed recipes, simple instructions, and practical tips to help you incorporate these herbal remedies into your routine.

Herbal Tea Blends for Digestion and Relaxation

Chamomile & Fennel Digestive Tea

Ingredients:

- 1 tsp dried chamomile flowers
- 1 tsp fennel seeds, lightly crushed
- 1 cup boiling water

Instructions:

1. Combine chamomile and fennel in a mug or small teapot.
2. Pour boiling water over the herbs and steep for 8–10 minutes.
3. Strain and sip slowly.

Lemon & Ginger Morning Spark Tea

Ingredients:

- Juice of ½ a lemon
- 1-inch fresh ginger root, sliced
- 1 cup water
- 1 tsp honey (optional)

Instructions:

1. Bring water and sliced ginger to a boil, then simmer for five minutes.
2. Strain into a cup and add lemon juice.
3. Sweeten with honey if desired.

Cinnamon-Spiced Digestive Aid

Ingredients:

- 1 cinnamon stick or 1 tsp ground cinnamon
- 1 tsp dried peppermint leaves
- 1 cup water

Instructions:

1. Boil the cinnamon in water for 5 minutes.
2. Add peppermint leaves and steep for another 5 minutes.
3. Strain and enjoy warm.

Lavender & Lemongrass Relaxation Blend

Ingredients:

- 1 tsp dried lavender flowers
- 1 stalk fresh lemongrass or 1 tsp dried lemongrass
- 1 cup boiling water

Instructions:

1. Combine lavender and lemongrass in a heatproof container.
2. Pour boiling water over the herbs and steep for 7–10 minutes.
3. Strain and sip slowly to relax.

Sorrel & Ginger Stress Relief Tea

Ingredients:

- 2 tbsp dried sorrel flowers
- 1-inch fresh ginger root, sliced
- 2 cups water
- 1 tsp brown sugar or honey

Instructions:

1. Boil sorrel and ginger in water for 10 minutes.
2. Strain the liquid and sweeten with brown sugar or honey.

Topical Applications for Skin Health

Oats & Aloe Calming Mask

Ingredients:

- 2 tbsp ground oats
- 2 tbsp fresh aloe vera gel
- 1 tsp honey

Instructions:

1. Mix all ingredients into a smooth paste.
2. Wash and dry your face, then apply the paste evenly.
3. Leave on for 15 minutes and rinse with lukewarm water.

Hydrating Coconut & Chamomile Balm

Ingredients:

- 2 tbsp coconut oil
- 1 tsp dried chamomile flowers

Instructions:

1. Melt coconut oil in a saucepan over low heat, then add chamomile flowers.
2. Simmer gently for 15 minutes, then strain into a clean jar.
3. Allow it to solidify, then apply as needed.

Neem Leaf Cleanser

Ingredients:

- 1 handful fresh neem leaves
- ½ cup water

Instructions:

1. Blend the neem leaves with water until smooth.
2. Apply to your face using a cotton ball or your fingers.
3. Leave for 10 minutes, then rinse.

Cooling Cucumber Mask

Ingredients:

- ½ cucumber, peeled and blended
- 2 tbsp plain yogurt

Instructions:

1. Mix cucumber puree with yogurt until smooth.
2. Apply evenly to your face and relax for 20 minutes.
3. Rinse with cool water.

Turmeric Healing Salve

Ingredients:

- 1 tsp turmeric powder
- 2 tbsp coconut oil
- ½ tsp beeswax

Instructions:

1. Melt coconut oil and beeswax in a double boiler, then stir in turmeric.
2. Pour into a small, sterilized jar and cool.

Remedies for Respiratory Support

Lemongrass & Basil Cold Tea

Ingredients:

- 1 stalk lemongrass, crushed
- 4 fresh basil leaves
- 2 cups water

Instructions:

1. Boil lemongrass and basil leaves in water for 10 minutes.
2. Strain and serve warm.

Turmeric Milk (Golden Milk)

Ingredients:

- 1 cup milk (dairy or non-dairy)
- 1 tsp turmeric powder
- ½ tsp cinnamon powder
- 1 tsp honey

Instructions:

1. Warm the milk and stir in turmeric and cinnamon.
2. Sweeten with honey to taste.

Peppermint & Licorice Root Steam

Ingredients:

- 1 tsp dried peppermint
- 1 tsp licorice root
- 3 cups boiling water

Instructions:

1. Add herbs to a large bowl, then pour over boiling water.
2. Cover your head with a towel and inhale steam deeply.

Homemade Thyme Vapor Rub

Ingredients:

- 1 tbsp coconut oil
- 1 tsp beeswax
- 5 drops thyme essential oil

Instructions:

1. Melt the coconut oil and beeswax over low heat.
2. Add the drops of thyme oil, stir, and store in a small jar.

Moringa & Ginger Respiratory Boost Tea

Ingredients:

- 1 tsp dried moringa leaves
- 1 slice fresh ginger
- 2 cups water

Instructions:

1. Boil moringa and ginger in water for 5–7 minutes.
2. Strain and drink warm or cool.

Integrating Herbal Remedies with Modern Medicine

The growing interest in herbal remedies has encouraged many people to explore natural healing alongside modern medical treatments. But how do you merge these two approaches responsibly and effectively? Integrating Jamaican herbal remedies with modern medicine requires education, open communication, and a balanced mindset.

This chapter will guide you through understanding potential interactions, speaking with your healthcare provider, and blending traditional and contemporary approaches for your health and well-being.

Understanding Interactions and Contraindications

Herbal remedies, while natural, are powerful tools for healing, and their active compounds can interact with medications or affect certain conditions. Common herbal remedies, such as turmeric, garlic, or ginger, can influence the way your body processes drugs. To safely integrate herbal treatments into your routine, you must first understand their potential effects.

Key Considerations

1. ***Drug-Herb Interactions***: Some herbs can increase or decrease the potency of medications you're taking. For example, St. John's Wort, a popular herb for mood support, can reduce the effectiveness of medications such as birth control pills, antidepressants, or blood thinners. Similarly, ginger may thin the blood, which could pose risks if you're already taking anticoagulant medications.
2. ***Dosages Matter***: Herbal remedies, like modern drugs, are potent in specific quantities. Taking an excessive dose can lead to side effects, while too little may reduce the remedy's efficacy. The "more is better" mindset does not work with herbal medicine.
3. ***Preexisting Conditions***: If you have conditions like diabetes, high blood pressure, or kidney disease, some herbs may exacerbate symptoms or interfere with treatment. For instance, ginseng may raise blood pressure levels, so it might not be suitable for someone with hypertension.
4. ***Allergies and Sensitivities***: Always ensure you're not allergic to a specific herb before using it. Test a small amount first, especially when applying topically, to avoid adverse reactions.

Actionable Steps

- Research the herbs you're interested in to learn about their known interactions.
- Use reputable sources like books written by herbal medicine experts or consult a trained herbalist.
- Start small; incorporate one remedy at a time to monitor its effects on your body while avoiding confusion about which herb might be causing side effects.

Communicating with Healthcare Providers

Maintaining open lines of communication with your doctor or other healthcare professionals is essential to safely integrating herbal remedies into your wellness plan. While some may be unfamiliar with Jamaican herbal traditions, a respectful and proactive conversation can help integrate their expertise with your goals.

How to Bring It Up

1. ***Be Honest and Transparent***: Tell your healthcare provider about all herbs or supplements you're taking. Even seemingly benign herbs like mint or chamomile can interact with certain medications, and your doctor needs this context to provide safe recommendations.
2. ***Use Clear Descriptions***: Share details about the specific herbs, doses, and your reasons for using them. For example, explain that you're using soursop leaf tea

to promote relaxation and minimize stress-related sleep disruptions.
3. *Ask Specific Questions*: Seek advice about whether the herb will interfere with your medications or treatment plan. For instance, if you're taking medication for inflammatory conditions, clarify if herbs like turmeric are safe to include.
4. *Accept Guidance*: Your doctor may caution you against certain herbs or combinations due to safety concerns. Trust their training and explore alternative remedies if necessary.

Tips for Building Productive Conversations

- Take notes during appointments and bring a list of questions or herbal remedies you're considering.
- If your doctor dismisses herbal remedies entirely or lacks knowledge, consider consulting a naturopath or integrative medicine specialist who bridges natural and conventional healthcare approaches.

By fostering these conversations, you take a team approach to your health, ensuring safety while pursuing a comprehensive blend of natural and modern techniques.

Combining Traditional and Contemporary Approaches

Merging herbal remedies with modern medicine is not about choosing one over the other; it's about creating a partnership between tradition and science. This balance can maximize the benefits of both worlds while minimizing risks.

Key Principles of Integration

1. ***Complement, Don't Replace***: Herbal remedies should support, not replace, prescribed treatments unless recommended by a healthcare provider. For example, using moringa tea to boost nutrient intake can complement medication for anemia but should not replace it without professional advice.
2. ***Use Both Therapies Strategically***: For chronic conditions like arthritis, you can pair anti-inflammatory medications with topical remedies like turmeric-infused oils to target swelling locally while managing systemic inflammation.
3. ***Target Specific Needs***: Choose remedies that fill gaps in your treatment plan. For instance, if stress management isn't fully addressed by your current medical plan, relaxation teas made with Jamaican herbs like lemongrass or soursop can provide additional support.

4. ***Regular Monitoring***: Monitor how your body reacts to combined treatments, like pairing aloe vera gel with prescribed ointments for improved wound healing.

Actionable Steps

- Create a log or journal to document the herbs and treatments you're using together, any positive changes, and any new symptoms or reactions.
- Experiment with timing to avoid overlapping doses. For example, take herbal teas at least an hour after medications unless instructed otherwise.
- Stay flexible; if one combination doesn't work, revisit your plan with your healthcare provider or herbal expert to find alternatives.

Blending herbal remedies with modern medicine creates balance between tradition and science. By understanding interactions, communicating with healthcare providers, and balancing therapies, you can achieve improved well-being holistically.

Growing Your Own Medicinal Herbs

Grow your own Jamaican medicinal herbs for fresh, potent remedies and a deeper connection to nature. This chapter provides tips on starting a home herb garden, caring for your plants, and preserving them for long-term use.

Tips for Starting a Home Herb Garden

Starting your herb garden is simpler than you might think. With the right planning and a little effort, you can cultivate a healthy, vibrant garden that provides access to fresh remedies year-round.

1. **Choose Your Herbs Wisely**

    Select herbs that suit your wellness goals and thrive in your local climate. Some versatile herbs to begin with include mint, lemongrass, basil, ginger, and turmeric, all staples in Jamaican herbal traditions.

    Example Starter Herbs and Their Benefits:

- *Mint*: Relieves nausea, aids digestion, and soothes stress.
- *Basil*: Acts as a natural anti-inflammatory and supports respiratory health.
- *Turmeric*: Fights inflammation and boosts overall immunity.

2. **Start Small**

Rather than planting a large variety, begin with 3–5 herbs to keep things manageable. You can grow these in pots or containers if you have limited space or directly in the ground if you have a garden area.

3. **Pick the Right Location**

Medicinal herbs generally need a good amount of sunlight to thrive. Look for a spot that gets 6–8 hours of direct sunlight daily. If you only have indoor space, place pots near a sunny window. Grow lights can also help if natural light is scarce.

4. **Invest in Quality Seeds and Starter Plants**

To ensure strong, healthy plants, purchase high-quality seeds or starter plants from trusted sources. Farmer's markets and local nurseries often have a good selection of herbs suited to your region.

5. **Use Companion Planting**

   Pair herbs that support each other's growth and resist pests naturally. For example, planting basil near mint can repel insects while creating a harmonious growing environment.

Beginner Tip: If you're unsure where to start, consider growing herbs in simple containers, like old pots or wooden boxes. This method makes them portable and easy to care for while you become familiar with their habits.

Soil, Climate, and Care Requirements

Caring for your herbs goes beyond planting them in soil. Follow these steps to provide the right environment and nutrients your herbs need to thrive.

1. *Soil Preparation*: The foundation of any garden is the soil. For most medicinal herbs, rich, well-draining soil is ideal. Herbs like basil and mint flourish in soil with good organic content.

   Steps for Preparing Soil:

   - Test your soil for pH (aim for a slightly acidic to neutral range, around 6.0–7.0).
   - Add compost or natural fertilizers like manure to enrich the soil.
   - Ensure proper drainage by loosening the soil or adding sand for clay-heavy areas.

2. ***Climate Considerations***: Many Jamaican herbs enjoy warm, tropical climates, but with care, they can adapt to other environments.

   Herb and Climate Examples:

   - Lemongrass: Thrives in hot, sunny climates and is sensitive to frost. Can grow in pots indoors in colder regions.
   - Ginger: Prefers warm and humid conditions. Can be grown in shaded spots outdoors or in a warm kitchen.
   - Mint: Adaptable and grows well even in mildly cool climates but needs regular watering.

3. ***Watering Practices***: Overwatering is a common mistake. Most herbs enjoy slightly moist soil but dislike sitting in water.

   Watering Tips:

   - Water deeply but less frequently to encourage strong root growth.
   - Check the top inch of soil daily; water only if it feels dry.
   - Use pots with drainage holes when growing in containers to prevent waterlogging.

4. ***Day-to-Day Care***: Medicinal herbs are relatively low-maintenance but respond well to care.

- Remove weeds regularly to prevent them from competing with your herbs for nutrients.
- Prune vigorously to encourage bushy growth and prevent plants from going to seed too early.

Beginner Tip: Start a garden journal! This can help you track what works best for each herb, especially in different seasons. Write down when you water or fertilize and note how your plants respond to changes.

Harvesting and Preserving Techniques

Once your herbs flourish, harvesting becomes one of the most satisfying aspects of gardening. Knowing when and how to harvest ensures that you reap their full medicinal benefits.

1. *Timing is Everything*: It's important to pick herbs at their peak for maximum potency. Here are some guidelines for common plants:
    - Mint and Basil: Harvest leaves early in the morning when the essential oils are most concentrated.
    - Ginger and Turmeric: Wait until the plants are mature, typically 8–10 months after planting.
    - Lemongrass: Harvest the outer stalks once they are thick and pale green.
2. *Harvesting Without Harming the Plant*: Careful harvesting ensures you can enjoy multiple yields from a single plant.

- Use sharp scissors or pruning shears to cut stems or leaves cleanly.
- Avoid harvesting more than 1/3 of the plant in a single session to allow recovery.

3. ***Drying Herbs for Long-Term Use***: Drying preserves your harvest so you can enjoy remedies year-round.

Air Drying:

- Cut small bunches of herbs and tie them together with string.
- Hang upside down in a well-ventilated, dark space.
- Once crisp, remove the dried leaves and store them in airtight jars.

Using a Dehydrator:

- Arrange clean herbs in a single layer on the dehydrator trays.
- Dry at a low temperature (95°F–115°F) for 1–4 hours, checking periodically.
- Store in sealed containers in a cool, dry place.

4. ***Preserving Freshness***: Fresh herbs leave a stronger impact. To keep herbs fresh longer, try these methods:
    - ***Freezing***: Chop herbs like mint or basil, place them in an ice cube tray, add water, and freeze. Use herb cubes in teas, soups, or remedies.

- ***Infused Oils***: Steep your herbs in olive oil or coconut oil to extract their active compounds for topical or culinary use.
5. ***Label and Rotate Stock***: To avoid wasting your hard-earned harvest, label your jars or packages with the date of preservation. Use older batches first to ensure nothing expires.

Growing medicinal herbs lets you create your own supply of natural remedies while fostering a deeper connection with nature. With care and patience, your herb garden can become a healing sanctuary, supporting your health whenever needed.

Resources and Further Reading

If you're ready to deepen your understanding of herbal remedies and how to incorporate them into your lifestyle, there are many great resources to guide you. From books and websites to workshops and courses, these tools will help you build both confidence and knowledge.

Recommended Books

Books on herbal medicine allow you to explore the topic in detail and at your own pace. Below are some excellent suggestions to get you started. Many of these books are available online, at libraries, or in bookstores.

1. ***"The Herbal Medicine-Maker's Handbook" by James Green***: A practical guide packed with hands-on techniques to prepare teas, tinctures, oils, and salves. It's perfect for anyone who wants to experiment with making their own herbal remedies.

    Here's the link to the book: https://tinyurl.com/bddd9sjs.

2. ***"Rosemary Gladstar's Herbal Recipes for Vibrant Health" by Rosemary Gladstar***: This beginner-friendly book offers simple recipes for a range of herbal preparations with a focus on wellness for the whole family.

   Here's the link to the book: https://tinyurl.com/yc43kjp6.

3. ***"Adaptogens: Herbs for Strength, Stamina, and Stress Relief" by David Winston and Steven Maimes***: A great choice if you're curious about herbs that help the body adapt to stress and improve resilience.

   Here's the link to the book: https://tinyurl.com/mr9y39af.

4. ***"Medical Herbalism" by David Hoffmann***: A more in-depth and technical resource for those interested in the science behind herbal medicine. This book provides a great foundation for advanced learning.

   Here's the link to the book: https://tinyurl.com/3mtrrt8s.

Pro Tip: Visit your local bookstore or library and ask for recommendations in the herbal or alternative medicine section. Don't forget second-hand bookshops; they often have hidden gems!

Trusted Websites

The internet is an incredible resource, but it's important to rely on trustworthy, science-backed websites. Here are some to consider:

- *American Herbalists Guild (AHG)*: A professional association for herbalists offering resources like informative articles, webinars, and directories to connect with certified practitioners.

  Here's the website link: https://americanherbalistsguild.com/.

- *Mountain Rose Herbs Blog*: This site not only sells high-quality herbs but also provides educational content on making herbal preparations and their benefits.

  Here's the website link: https://blog.mountainroseherbs.com/.

- *Herbal Academy Blog*: A fantastic source for beginner-friendly guides and advanced studies. Their articles often include recipes you can try at home.

  Here's the website link: https://theherbalacademy.com/.

- *NIH's National Center for Complementary and Integrative Health (NCCIH)*: A government resource providing evidence-based information about herbs and supplements.

Here's the website link: https://www.nccih.nih.gov/.

Tip for Exploration: When searching online, use keywords like "herbal medicine beginner tips" or "trusted herbal remedy guides" to find more resources.

Local and Online Suppliers

If you're making your own herbal preparations, sourcing high-quality herbs is crucial. Here's how to find the best suppliers:

- *Local Health Food Stores and Co-ops*: These stores often carry loose herbs, pre-mixed teas, and natural products. Talk to the staff, as they can usually provide great advice.
- *Farmers' Markets*: Local growers may have fresh chamomile, lavender, or other seasonal herbs. Building relationships with farmers ensures you're getting organic, locally sourced products.
- *Online Retailers*: Companies like Mountain Rose Herbs, Starwest Botanicals, and Frontier Co-op are well-known for their organic and ethically sourced herbs. Order in bulk to save money and stock your home apothecary.

Pro Tip: Before buying online, check reviews for the company and ensure products are certified organic or wild-harvested when possible.

Workshops and Courses on Herbal Medicine

Taking part in workshops and courses is one of the best ways to deepen your knowledge of herbal remedies. Many courses are designed for beginners, so don't worry if you're just getting started.

- *Local Workshops*: Check community bulletin boards, health food stores, or local herbalists' clinics for announcements. Public gardens and botanical centers often host herbal medicine classes too.
- *Online Courses*: Platforms such as Herbal Academy, Chestnut School of Herbal Medicine, or LearningHerbs offer comprehensive beginner and advanced courses. Topics range from herbal DIY projects to in-depth studies of plant properties. Courses often include videos, PDFs, and group discussions.
- *Herbalist Certifications*: For those looking to pursue a deeper and professional understanding, many schools offer certification programs. These programs typically cover in-depth plant biology, herbal formulation, and safety. Search for programs accredited by the American Herbalists Guild.

With these resources, you'll be well on your way to becoming more knowledgeable and confident with using herbal remedies in your daily life. Whether it's through books, blogs, hands-on workshops, or finding high-quality herbal suppliers, expanding your understanding will support your wellness journey.

Conclusion

Thank you for taking the time to read through this comprehensive guide on Jamaican herbal medicine. By doing so, you've taken an important step in exploring a remarkable tradition that blends the wisdom of culture, the healing properties of nature, and the principles of holistic health. Learning about this practice not only deepens your appreciation for herbal remedies but also empowers you to make more intentional choices for your well-being.

Jamaican herbal medicine offers immense value because of its accessibility, sustainability, and effectiveness. It's a practice rooted in history, yet highly relevant in today's wellness-focused world. At its core, these remedies emphasize prevention and balance, teaching us that health involves nurturing the body, mind, and spirit in harmony. Whether you're looking to address specific ailments, strengthen your immune system, or simply reconnect with nature, this tradition provides a wealth of resources and practices that can benefit your daily life.

You've learned that Jamaican herbs like ginger, turmeric, and soursop are more than just plants; they are tools for self-care and healing. The act of using them draws you closer to the natural world and reminds you of the beauty in simple, mindful living. By incorporating these remedies into your routine, you're not just supporting your own health but also honoring a practice rooted in ancestral knowledge and respect for nature's gifts.

Now that you've explored the depth and richness of this tradition, the next step is putting it into action. Start small and choose one or two remedies that resonate with you. Maybe it's as simple as brewing a calming soursop tea in the evening or growing a pot of mint on your windowsill. These small efforts will allow you to build confidence while establishing a deeper connection to the benefits of herbal medicine.

Remember, your journey with herbal remedies doesn't have to be perfect. You don't need to know everything to begin. It's okay to experiment, adapt, and learn as you go. If questions arise, seek guidance. Turn to trusted herbalists, reliable books, or workshops to expand your knowledge. And always listen to your body. Pay attention to how it responds, and make adjustments to find what works best for you. Approach this process as a partnership with nature, one that evolves over time.

Beyond the physical benefits, you may find that this practice opens doors to self-reflection, mindfulness, and sustainable habits. Growing your own herbs, preparing your own remedies, or simply sipping a homemade tea can foster a sense of accomplishment and peace. It reminds you that wellness is not just a quick fix but a lifelong commitment to balance, care, and intentional living.

Thank you for exploring Jamaican herbal medicine. You're now equipped to deepen your journey, whether by learning more, integrating remedies with modern medicine, or connecting with nature. Embrace curiosity and intention as you continue your path toward health and well-being.

FAQs

Are Jamaican herbal remedies safe to use?

Yes, Jamaican herbal remedies are generally safe when used correctly, but it's essential to approach them with care. Start by researching the herbs you plan to use, follow appropriate dosages, and consult a professional if you have underlying health conditions or are taking medications. Pregnant or breastfeeding individuals should exercise additional caution.

Where can I find high-quality Jamaican herbs?

High-quality Jamaican herbs can be found at local farmers' markets, herbal shops, or through reputable online suppliers. Look for organic or sustainably sourced options, and avoid herbs with unnatural additives. If possible, build a relationship with trusted vendors or consider growing your own herbs for guaranteed freshness.

Can I combine Jamaican herbal remedies with modern medicine?

Yes, but it's important to be cautious. Certain herbs can interact with medications, either strengthening or reducing their effects. Always consult your healthcare provider before combining herbal remedies with prescribed treatments to ensure safety and compatibility.

How can I start incorporating herbal remedies into my routine?

Begin by identifying your health goals, such as improving digestion or reducing stress. Start with one or two simple remedies, like herbal teas, tinctures, or salves, and pair them with existing habits, such as drinking tea during your morning ritual. Gradually add more remedies as you become comfortable with their use.

Do herbal remedies work immediately?

Some remedies, like calming teas, may show noticeable results within minutes or hours, offering quick relief from stress and anxiety. Others, however, such as remedies designed to boost immunity or improve digestion, often require weeks of consistent use to deliver significant benefits.

This is because herbal remedies typically work by supporting and gradually restoring balance to your body's natural systems rather than providing an immediate fix. Consistency and patience are essential when using these remedies, as their true effectiveness often lies in long-term use and integration into your daily routine.

Can I grow Jamaican herbs at home?

Absolutely! Many Jamaican herbs like mint, ginger, and lemongrass thrive in common garden conditions or even in pots. They need well-draining soil, adequate sunlight, and regular care. Growing your own herbs ensures you have fresh, chemical-free ingredients for your remedies.

What are the most versatile Jamaican herbs to start with?

Begin with staples like ginger (for digestion and colds), turmeric (for inflammation), mint (for nausea and stress relief), and soursop leaves (for relaxation). These herbs are easy to use in teas and other remedies and provide a wide range of health benefits.

References and Helpful Links

The Master Guide to Jamaican Herbal Remedies: Discovering Health and Harmony with Natural Jamaican Herbs: Lewis, Tafari: 9798313654560: Amazon.com: Books. (n.d.).
https://www.amazon.com/Master-Guide-Jamaican-Herbal-Remedies/dp/B0F13LYW8B

Tea, S. |. O. +. S. (2024, February 6). Jamaican herbs that you should always keep on hand + Remedies. Orchids + Sweet Tea.
https://www.orchidsandsweettea.com/jamaican-herbs-that-you-should-always-keep-on-hand-remedies/

Lifestyle, Y. (2020, June 29). 10 Best Jamaican herbs for respiratory health and immune support. Yaga Lifestyle.
https://yagalifestyle.com/blogs/jamaican-herbs/10-best-jamaican-herbs-for-respiratory-health-and-immune-support?srsltid=AfmBOoqZ7EcFNNhDRQ71M65D-cIftngRC2qGQD6pohPsCf26tbKS6ZJ1

Summerfield Books. (2019, October 13). Jamaican Herbs And Medicinal Plants And Their Uses from Summerfield Books.
https://www.summerfieldbooks.com/product/jamaican-herbs-and-medicinal-plants-and-their-uses/

Healing Jamaica: Exploring the rich tradition of plant medicine. (2025, March 5). Croydon in the Mountains.
https://www.croydon-estate.com/healing-jamaica-tradition-of-plant-medicine

Thiele, J. (2024, August 28). A beginner's guide to growing medicinal herbs | Western herbal medicine | Herbal Reality. Herbal Reality. https://www.herbalreality.com/herbalism/western-herbal-medicine/beginner-guide-growing-medicinal-herbs/

Doctor, S. S. N. (n.d.). Forms of herbs / Botanicals. https://www.naturesintentionsnaturopathy.com/botanical-medicine/botanical-essentials.html

www.ingramcontent.com/pod-product-compliance
Lightning Source LLC
LaVergne TN
LVHW012029060526
838201LV00061B/4528